Ba

Cookbook for Gastric Bypass

Easy and Healthy Recipes to Enjoy Favorite Foods Before and After Weight-Loss Surgery

Mike Basso

Disclaimer

TABLE OF CONTENTS

4

Introduction

Undergoing gastric bypass surgery is one of the biggest decisions you can make in your life. This surgery is known for its high success rate as well as the fast rate at which it works. However, similar to most things in life, its actual success depends on how much you know about it and how well prepared you are for it. The gastric bypass surgery is not a piece of cake. If you've decided to go through it, you'll need all the help you can get as well as some determination. Luckily, you have this book and with the right motivation and steadfastness, your gastric bypass surgery will be a success from start to finish.

A lot of people believe that the surgery simply takes off excess weight and that it requires nothing else. While it is true that the surgery takes off weight, you should know that with poor eating habits, you could end up worse-off or back at square one. This would be wasted time, effort, and money. If you stick to the recipes and meal plan in this book diligently, you'll be on your way to a healthier and better life. Welcome to the gastric bypass surgery club.

Gastric bypass surgery and your diet

How does gastric bypass affect the diet?

The biggest thing affected by the gastric bypass surgery is the diet. Weeks after the surgery, the human body heals completely from it and so the pains and most discomforts will fade away. What won't fade away is how you have to have a new approach to food. You will literally never look at food the same way again. This surgery is like initiating you into a new way of looking at food. From compulsive eating and simply eating whenever you feel like, you'll move to eating exactly what your body eats and nothing more. This change is something that begins from the moment you make your decision to get a gastric bypass surgery.

Pre-op gastric bypass surgery diet

Your diet changes as early as 3 weeks before your operation. We refer to this diet as the pre-op diet. Your diet changes earlier mainly because of the surgery. The diet mainly consists of foods that are low in fat and sugar. When you eat approved and safe foods, it makes the surgery move much safely and easily for the doctor and you. The fatty foods which you consume would be cut down on. When you cut down on them, the fat around the liver is reduced. When that happens, doctors can get smoother access to your stomach during the surgery. That way, the risk of complications is reduced. An obese person has a higher risk of complications during surgery. Since the diet is a bit of what your post-op diet will be, it'll help you get ready for the change in diet plans after the surgery.

During the three weeks before the gastric bypass surgery, you are expected to cut down on calories. In a bid to do this, you must cut down on your intake of carbs. A lot of the carbs we take in have high levels of calories. You are also expected to cut down on your intake of unhealthy fats. Of course not all fats are bad or unhealthy. This is why fats are clearly divided into the healthy and unhealthy segment. You will need to stop all unhealthy fats and focus on the healthy fats. You will also need to increase your intake of proteins. Proteins should be what you consume the most. Before your surgery, you should develop the habit of counting calories before you eat. Start now to develop a habit. Another important thing is to keep your hydration levels really high. Drink clean and fresh water and stop soft drinks and alcohol.

Three days before your gastric surgery, you will need to begin your all-liquid diet. You are not going to consume any solids within this period. Whatever liquids you take must be healthy. You can heave low-calorie *energy drinks for sports*. However, you must not take soft drinks or alcohol.

On the midnight of the day of your surgery, you must take nothing at all. If your surgery is scheduled for 2PM on a *Thursday*, you must stop eating immediately it gets to 11:59pm on *Wednesday*. If you don't do this, the doctors will not operate on you if you tell them. If you do not tell them and you choose to go on with the surgery, serious complications and even death could occur.

Post-op gastric bypass surgery diet

The moment the surgery is completed, your new diet begins in full force. The aim of the diet is to help you recover in the best way possible. The gastric bypass diet comes in various stages. Each stage shows that you are healing a little bit more. As you progress, you can go a little higher in your gastric bypass surgery diet. For easy remembering, the gastric bypass surgery has been divided into 5 stages. These stages do not include the pre-op diet. They are simply for the post-op diet.

Stage 1- Clear liquids
The first stage includes only liquids. This stage starts after the surgery. For about 1-7 days after the surgery, the patient can take only clear liquids. Your dietician will let you know exactly how long to stay in this stage.

Stage 2A-Full liquid
This diet includes full liquids. Full liquids are semi-liquid and are not see-through. It is midway between clear liquids and pureed foods. Here, your liquids can start to have some chunks of solid foods. This stage lasts for 1-2 weeks

Stage 2B- Pureed foods
After that stage, this next one lasts for 1-2 weeks. Here, you can consume liquid forms of protein. You should be taking up to 70 grams of protein and 64 ounces of fluids.

Stage 3- Soft foods
In this stage, patients can begin to eat soft foods that can be easily mashed. You should be taking up to 70 grams of protein and 64 ounces of clear water. You should also eat about 1-2 ounces in each serving. You should also take a very little portion of healthy fats. Usually, this comes from an avocado.

Stage 4- Solid foods
Here you can go back to eating solid foods. This diet starts from that point to the rest of your life. You should eat mainly protein and vegetables. The grains you consume should be in limited quantities. Your intake of sugar should be at the barest minimum. This will be your stage for the rest of your life.

Dos and don'ts of gastric bypass surgery diet
As expected, there are some things you are simply not allowed to do when it comes to your gastric bypass diet. Here are some of them.

1. No straw- This applies from stage 1 to stage 3. You should not use straws to take in your liquids. This is because using straws can take in unwanted air into the stomach.
2. Do not eat more than one new food per day- Your body will have different reactions to new foods even though you have eaten them before the surgery. Anything you haven't eaten after the surgery is a new food. Do not try more than one per day.
3. Learn how to chew- The way that you used to chew before the surgery is no longer the way you will chew. Before, chewing was a careless thing we did. However, now, you must learn how to chew again. Time yourself to ensure that you chew each bite for as long as 15-seconds.
4. Drink water- At stage four, drink at least 64 ounces of water each day. Take water 30 minutes after food.
5. Avoid processed carbs and sugar- Stay away from foods that have high levels of sugar and refined or processed carbohydrates
6. Stay away from unhealthy fats- Make sure you avoid foods that have unhealthy fat.
7. Learn how to eat- Learn to chew proteins first. When they are eaten, eat your vegetables, and then carbohydrates.

Food cravings after gastric surgery

After your gastric bypass surgery you may find that you encounter a lot of cravings. It is only natural and you can be assured that after some time, your body will adjust and you will have few cravings. In case you have cravings, here are some tips to help you manage them.

1. Invest in healthy snacks- Purchase healthy snacks. When you purchase healthy snacks, you can have them when you are hungry to take your mind off food cravings.
2. Do not skip meals- To succeed in this diet, you must find balance. Finding your balance involves eating when you should and when you shouldn't. Skipping one meal can put in discord to your hard work as your stomach is now extremely sensitive.
3. Drink water- In a day, ensure you have as much as 8 glasses. When you are craving, take a big gulp or two.
4. Plan your environments- Do not go to a fast food restaurant where everyone will be eating what you can't eat. Plan your environments. Plan where you are supposed to stay.
5. Distract yourself- Distracting yourself when you are cravings will help you out. Get up and do something you like.

A new way to eat

Gastric surgery proposes a new way to eat. From relearning and reintroducing food to new time tables and even to new ways to chew, you have to learn all these. Do not be too impatient with yourself. If your body doesn't like a particular food, dump it. Listen to your body and go at its pace. Remember to see your dietician frequently and express your struggles honestly.

Pre-op meal plan

At this point, you will begin to eat 5 times a day. You will have one meal, two protein shakes [one for each period], and two no-sugar snacks [one for each period]. You should eat them in this order:

1. Breakfast- *One* protein shake
2. Mid morning- *One* vegetable or fruit-based snack. You can also have a fruit that has 150- 250 calories
3. Lunch/ Dinner *One* main meal
4. Evening *One* protein shake
5. Lunch/ Dinner *One* vegetable or fruit-based snack

Note that you can have those meals in any order but you must space them out. You must consume at least 64 ounces or 8 cups of any sugar-free beverage such as water or sugar-free sport drinks.

Allowed liquids are-

- Water
- Decaf coffee or coffee substitute and tea
- Fruit flavored drinks
- Clear broth
- Clear juices (grape, cranberry, and apple)
- Smooth fruit ices or popsicles
- Gelatins

On a total, for the pre-op diet women may consume about 1200 calories while men may consume about 1500 calories. You can

Suggestions for protein shakes

Here are some suggestions for protein shakes. Note that whatever protein shake you want to take should have the following nutritional values per serving:

- Protein- 15-25+ grams
- Added sugar- less than 7 grams
- Calories- 100-250
- Total fat- 4 grams and below
- A short list of added ingredients
- They must be made from 100% whey protein isolate or whey protein

Here are some examples of such brands:

- Costc Premium Protein Shakes
- GNC Pure Protein Shakes
- World Wide Protein Shakes

Suggestions for snacks

Here are some suggestions for snacks. Note that whatever protein shake you want to take should have the following nutritional values per serving:

- Protein- 15-25+ grams
- Added sugar- less than 7 grams
- Calories- 100-250
- Total fat- 4 grams and below
- A short list of added ingredients

Protein Shake is ideal

Alternatively, you could take another protein shake. Here are some snacks you can take.

- 1 Protein bar [the options are numerous]
- 1 boiled egg
- Protein pre-made drinks

- Diet yoghurt
- 2 rice cakes
- 5-6 crackers with 1 ounce of low fat cheese
- 5 ounces of strawberries
- ½ English muffin
- ¼ cup of unsalted nuts
- 1 cup of starch-free vegetables and 1 tablespoon of salad dressing
- 1 serving of fruit 150-250 calories
- ½ cup of low fat cottage cheese

If you rotate these options, they would suit for 2-3 weeks.

Note that you should give a 30 minutes gap between food and liquid.

Pre-op main meals for gastric surgery

1. Cream of wheat hot cereal

NUTRITIONAL VALUE PER SERVING

Carbs: 78; Calories: 369; Total Fat: 0.5g; Protein: 11g; Sugar: 0g

Servings: 1

Preparation time: 10 minutes

Ingredients:

- 2 tablespoons of cream of wheat cereal
- 1 cup of skimmed milk
- Pinch of salt

Directions

- In a small bowl, pour in your cream of wheat
- Next, pour in your milk and stir well.
- Pour the mix in a saucepan and bring to boil on a low heat for 5 minutes.
- Turn the fire off and add a pinch of salt.
- Stir thoroughly and serve warm.

2. Chicken breast fillets and peppers
NUTRITIONAL VALUE PER SERVING

Carbs: 10.6; Calories: 211; Total Fat: 3.3g; Protein: 28.1g; Sugar: 0g

Servings: 1

Preparation time: 45 minutes

Ingredients:

- 1 skinless and boneless chicken
- ½ tablespoon of olive oil
- 1 small sliced onions
- Pinch of salt
- Pinch of thyme
- 1 small red pepper, diced
- 1 small tomato, diced

- ¼ teaspoon of grounded pepper

- 1 teaspoon of chopped parsley
- ¼ teaspoon of chopped oregano
- Low fat cooking spray

Directions

- Pour oil in skillet and heat at medium
- Stir fry till soft
- Pour in red peppers and stir fry
- When they are soft, put in tomatoes
- Add seasonings such as salt, thyme, grounded pepper, oregano, and parsley
- Stir fry for 5 minutes and take off heat and cover
- Spray cooking oil generously in dry pan
- Place chicken in pan and cook on medium heat

16

- Cook for three minutes on each side
- Take out the fried chicken and place in covered pan with tomatoes and pepper
- Place on fire and cook for three minutes
- Serve hot or warm

3. Lean Hamburgers
NUTRITIONAL VALUE PER SERVING

Carbs: 8; Calories: 200; Total Fat: 9g; Protein: 25g; Sugar: 0g; Cholesterol: 60mg; Potassium: 290mg

Servings: 1

Preparation time: 40 minutes

Ingredients:

- ¼ pound 95 percent of ground lean beef
- ½ chopped onion
- ½ tablespoon of Worcestershire sauce
- Pinch of salt
- ¼ teaspoon of grounded pepper
- 1 tablespoon of canola oil
- *low carb* hamburger bun

Directions

- Heat oil in skillet on medium heat
- Pour in onions and stir fry till soft
- Take off heat and allow cool
- When slightly cool, pour in ground beef, pinch of salt and pepper
- Stir and pour mixture in bowl
- From it, form a single patty. Make sure it is pressed together and firm
- Place the patty in a grill for 11 to 15 minutes on medium heat
- Place fried patty in low carb hamburger bun

4. Meatballs
NUTRITIONAL VALUE PER SERVING

Carbs: 8; Calories: 200; Total Fat: 10g; Protein: 22.1g; Sugar: 0g; Fibers: 2.1g

Servings: 1

Preparation time: 40 minutes

Ingredients:

- ¼ pound of ground lean beef
- 1/8 cup of fine, dry breadcrumbs
- 1/8 cup milk
- Freshly ground black pepper
- 1 small egg
- 1 tablespoon fresh parsley leaves
- ½ teaspoon of salt
- 1 small diced onion
- 1/8 teaspoon of minced garlic

Directions

- Rim baking sheet and preheat oven to 400°F
- Crack and mix egg
- In a bowl, pour in breadcrumbs and then milk. Stir and leave
- Mix pepper, parsley, and salt in another bowl. Pour in about half of the mixed egg
- Mix and pour in beef. Use your hands to mix very well
- Pour in the breadcrumbs mix
- Add onions and mix well
- Mold the mix into balls. You should have about 5
- Bake at 400°F for 20 to 25 minutes till very brown
- Serve hot

5. *Shrimp ceviche*
NUTRITIONAL VALUE PER SERVING

Calories: 160 kals; Fat: 1 gram; Cholesterol: 0.022 grams; Sodium: 0.265 grams; Carbohydrates: 13 grams; Dietary Fiber: 2 grams; Sugar: 5 grams; Protein: 25 grams.

Servings: 5 ounces per person

Preparation time: 30 minutes

Ingredients:

- 1 cup of fresh lime juice
- 1 pound of medium raw shrimp
- 3 small minced chili peppers (Serrano)
- 1 small onion (red) finely chopped (approx. ¾ cup chopped)
- 1 bunch cilantro, stemmed, chopped finely.
- 5 medium sized tomatoes, diced

Directions

- Wash shrimps thoroughly in clean water. Make sure that the water is at room temperature.
- Put in the shrimp into a medium sized bowl and pour the fresh lime juice into bowl as well
- Leave the shrimp to marinate (soak) in the lime until the color changes to pink. (This should take about 10 minutes). The shrimp must be marinated properly to produce the distinctive flavor.
- Add in your finely chopped onions, minced chili peppers, and diced tomatoes and cilantro. Stir gently to let the flavor circulate.
- Add salt to taste.
- Refrigerate for at least one hour and serve cold

6. *Baked chicken with vegetables*
NUTRITIONAL VALUE PER SERVING

Calories grams: 240 kals; Sugar: 9.998 grams; Carbohydrate: 25 grams, Protein: 26 grams; Fat: 3.5; Fibre: 4 grams; Sodium: 0.130 grams.

Servings: 5 ounces per person

Preparation time: 2 hours

Ingredients:

- 1½ cup water
- 3 finely sliced carrots,
- ½ of a large onion, (quartered)
- 2 potatoes,
- Raw chicken (cut into several pieces and remove all the top skin)
- 1 teaspoon of thyme
- ¼ teaspoon of pepper

Directions

- Wash, peel and Slice your potatoes
- Put the sliced potatoes, onions and carrots in a roasting pan
- Place pieces of raw chicken on top of the vegetables
- Then mix your teaspoon of thyme and quarter spoon of pepper together and mix with water.
- Pour this suspension over the chicken. It will sink to the vegetables below.
- Repeat this process once or twice during baking by spooning the suspension over the chicken and vegetables. This will enable the spices and seasoning to permeate the chicken adequately
- Leave to bake for 50 minutes at 425.

7. Oregano zucchini pizza and sauce
NUTRITIONAL VALUE PER SERVING

Calories: 100kal; protein 3.60g; Carbohydrate: 16.75g; Fat 1.25g.

Servings: 2 servings

Preparation time: 40 minutes

Ingredients:

Dough-

- Whole wheat tortilla flat bread
- One table spoon of pizza sauce
- One thinly sliced table spoon of zucchini
- 1 table spoon of grated pizza cheese (low fat)
- Tomatoes or mushrooms (optional)

Sauce-

- 1 can of tomato sauce
- ½ teaspoons of oregano
- 1 teaspoon of rosemary
- 1 teaspoon of thyme
- 2 scoops of unjury
- 2 minced onions
- 2 cloves of garlic

Directions

Dough-

- Fry the zucchini in a non-stick skillet sprayed with cooking spray. Do not take off until it is slightly browned
- Spread Tortilla with a small amount of Pizza sauce
- Sprinkle the zucchini with some cheese after placing it on the tortilla
- With your oven at a temperature of 360 degrees, bake until cheese melts (this should take approximately 22-25 minutes)

- Garnish by adding either sliced tomatoes or mushrooms

Sauce-

- In a non-stick skillet spray with extra virgin olive oil cooking spray, Saute' until tender and clear.
- Mix the onion, garlic, oregano, thyme, rosemary and unjury together.
- Pile the mixture on the crust
- Bake for 24 minutes in a 405 degree oven.

8. Baked salmon
NUTRITIONAL VALUE PER SERVING

Calories grams: 180 kals; Carbohydrate: 4 grams, Protein: 28 grams; Fat: 7; Fiber: 1 grams; Cholesterol: 60mg

Servings: 5 ounces per person

Preparation time: 35 minutes

Ingredients:

- 1 pound side of salmon without the skin
- 3 sprigs of rosemary
- 1/8 teaspoon of pepper
- 1 ½ tablespoon of olive oil
- 1 teaspoon of salt
- 1 small lemon thinly sliced
- 1 clove of chopped garlic

Directions

- Prepare baking sheet and line with aluminum foil and spray with baking spray
- Preheat oven to 375 degrees F
- Mix the oil, pepper, and salt
- Rub generously on salmon
- Place 1 ½ rosemary in the middle of the baking pan
- Place half of the lemon on the rosemary
- Place salmon on lemon and rosemary
- Place the garlic and remaining rosemary and lemon on it

9. Spaghetti and tomato sauce
NUTRITIONAL VALUE PER SERVING

Calories grams: 264 kals; Carbohydrate: 49 grams, Protein: 9.04 grams; Fat: 3.68

Servings: 5 ounces per person

Preparation time: 1 ½ hours

Ingredients:

- Plain spaghetti
- 2 pounds of ripe tomatoes
- 1 teaspoon of tomato paste
- 1 mashed garlic clove
- 1 spoon of virgin olive oil
- 2 pinches of salt
- ½ teaspoon pepper
- ½ small finely chopped onion

Directions

- Heat slightly salted water in a sauce pan.
- When boiling, pour in spaghetti
- Boil for 20-25 minutes and pour in strainer to take water out
- Pour back in pot and cover to keep warm
- Slice tomatoes and take out inner parts with seeds
- Grate the tomatoes with a hand grater or for 1 -3 seconds with a blender to give it a rough look
- In a skillet, heat oil at medium heat
- Put in onion and fry till soft
- Put in garlic and pepper and stir
- Pour in tomato paste and stir fry for a minute or two
- Put in tomato and add salt to taste
- Cover and let steam for 45 – 50 minutes
- Serve spaghetti with sauce

10. Shrimp alfredo
NUTRITIONAL VALUE PER SERVING

Calories grams: 422 kals; : 3.9 grams; Carbohydrate: 32.6 grams, Protein: 24.9 grams; Fat: 13.5; Sodium: 586.2 grams.

Servings: 5 ounces per person

Preparation time: 2 hours

Ingredients:

- 1½ cup water
- 3 finely sliced carrots,
- ½ of a large onion, (quartered)
- 2 potatoes,
- Raw chicken (cut into several pieces and remove all the top skin)
- 1 teaspoon of thyme
- ¼ teaspoon of pepper

Directions

- Wash, peel and Slice your potatoes
- Put the sliced potatoes, onions and carrots in a roasting pan
- Place pieces of raw chicken on top of the vegetables
- Then mix your teaspoon of thyme and quarter spoon of pepper together and mix with water.
- Pour this suspension over the chicken. It will sink to the vegetables below.
- Repeat this process once or twice during baking by spooning the suspension over the chicken and vegetables. This will enable the spices and seasoning to permeate the chicken adequately
- Leave to bake for 50 minutes at 425.

Sample meal plan for pre-op gastric bypass surgery

- 7:00- 8 ounces of water
- 8:00 am- 8:30am- Wide-world protein shake 1
- 9:00am- 8 ounces of decaf coffee
- 10:00am- 10:30am- 2 apples
- 11:00 am- 8 ounces of water
- 12:00pm-12:30pm- 2 servings of oregano zucchini pizza
- 1:00pm- 8 ounces of fruit flavored drinks
- 2:00- 8 ounces of clear broth
- 3:00- 8 ounces of plain gelatin
- 4:00pm- 4:30pm- 2 rice cakes
- 5:00pm- 8 ounces of water
- 6:30pm- GNc pure protein shake
- 7:00- 8 ounces of clear broth

This is a sample meal plan. Note that you should take your liquids 30 minutes after eating. Right now, since you haven't done the surgery, it isn't compulsory but after the surgery, it will be and so, it is better to get used to it. If you are really thirsty, just take a two-three sips of water.

You can also get into the habits of counting your calories so you can know how much of a particular non-starchy fruit you can take.

Remember to check calorie counts. If a serving has much more calories than you need, you can get half or a quarter.

Stage 1- Clear liquids meal plan

As we explained before, this stage kick starts immediately after the surgery. Once you are discharged from the hospital, your stomach needs to rest and heal from. You are expected to consume at least 70 grams of protein and 48 to 64 ounces of fluids. The protein and staying hydrated will help your body recover much faster.

You are expected to take liquids every two hours. You should not take more than two ounces at a go. This way, you do not rush your stomach and you can heal properly.

Stage 1- Clear liquids recipes

11. Italian chicken soup
NUTRITIONAL VALUE PER SERVING

Calories: 202.5kal; protein 15.8g; Carbohydrate: 20.6g; Fat 7g.

Preparation time: 40 minutes

Ingredients:

- 1 pound ground chicken
- Italian seasoned canned stewed tomatoes
- 1 can of rinsed and drained black beans
- ½ teaspoon fresh ground pepper
- 1 packet of Tofu
- 1 can of 99% fat free chicken
- ½ white onion
- ½ bay leaf
- 1 teaspoon salt
- 1 can of un-drained mixed vegetables
- 1 can of un-drained gold and white corn

Directions

- Mix bay leaf, broth and all the vegetables and season with salt and pepper
- Bring to a boil over low heat
- In a non-stick skillet, sauté onions until they become clear
- Add ground chicken, cook well and squeeze in a paper towel to remove all trace of fat
- Take chicken and Tofu and add to the cooking vegetables for about 10 minutes
- Garnish the meal with fresh Basil and baby spinach
- Boil for 30 minutes on low heat
- Strain to remove pieces of meat and vegetables

12. British clam broth
NUTRITIONAL VALUE PER SERVING

Calories: 97.2kal; protein 7.8g; Carbohydrate: 16.2g; Fat 7g

Preparation time: 30 minutes

Ingredients:

- ¼ teaspoon liquid smoke
- ¼ teaspoon pepper
- ¼ teaspoon salt
- 1 15 ounce can of evaporated milk (fat free)
- 1 15 ounce can of chicken broth (fat free)
- 1 medium sized fresh potato
- 1, 6 ounce can of undrained clams
- 1 bottle of clam juice (optional)

Directions

- Microwave your potato and chop it into smaller bits
- Mix it pepper, clam juice, milk, chicken broth, liquid smoke and season with salt
- Boil the mixture
- Dice the clams and add to the mixture
- Take off the fire immediately to prevent overcooking of the clams
- Season to taste with salt and pepper
- Boil on low heat for an hour
- Strain out to remove pieces of meat and vegetables

13. *Green pea chicken*

Calories: 120 kal; protein 13.4g; Carbohydrate: 14.4g; Fat 7g.

Preparation time:

Ingredients:

- 2 jars of baby green peas
- 4 tablespoons of sour cream (fat free)
- 2 spoons of chicken unjury
- 1/8 teaspoon of nutmeg
- 1/8 teaspoon of salt
- 1 cup half and half (fat free)

Directions

- Wash the fresh green baby peas
- Blend the peas , half and half, and nutmeg to a smooth consistency
- Pour into a cup and microwave for one minute.
- Allow to cool before pouring into blender with unjury chicken protein powder.
- Blend till veru smooth
- Place 2 spoonful's of fat free sour cream on the top before consumption
- Refrigerate to store

14. Baked potato soup
NUTRITIONAL VALUE PER SERVING

328 calories; 14.8 g total fat; 6.1 g saturated fat; 29 mg cholesterol; 400 mg sodium. 1023 mg potassium; 37.5 g carbohydrates; 2.7 g fiber; 2 g sugar; 14.1 g protein; 422

Preparation time: 50 mins

Ingredients:

1. 4 cups reduced-sodium chicken broth
2. 2 tablespoons canola oil
3. 1 large chopped onion
4. ¼ teaspoon freshly ground pepper
5. ½ cup reduced-fat sour cream
6. ½ cup shredded extra-sharp Cheddar cheese
7. 1 ½ pounds medium russet potatoes
8. 2 slices bacon

Directions

- Cut each slice of bacon in two
- Pour canola oil in large saucepan and heat on medium heat
- Put in the slices of bacon and fry on medium heat. Turn around until it is crisp. When it is fried and crisp, pick it out and put in paper towel to drain oil
- Put in the onions into the oil and stir fry till it is soft
- Pour in potatoes and broth and oil for 15 minutes
- Take potatoes out and blend them until they completely smooth. It should still have chunks
- Put the mashed potatoes back in the pot and pour in sour cream, cheese and pepper
- Boil for 3 minutes

15. Acorn Soup

NUTRITIONAL VALUE PER SERVING

Calories: 210g; Fat: 10g; Cholesterol: 1mg; Potassium:902mg; carbohydrates: 27g; 2.7 g fiber: 4g; sugar; 1.6g protein: 3.7g

Preparation time: 1 ½ hours

Ingredients:

- 1 large sliced onion
- 2 tablespoons of canola oil
- 1 ¼ cup of chicken broth
- 1 tablespoon of ground curry
- ¼ teaspoon of black pepper
- 3 acorn squashes
- 2 tablespoons of olive oil

Directions

- Cut each acorn squash in half and seed
- Preheat oven to 400 degrees F
- Line a baking sheet and placed it acorns face down on it
- Mix olive oil with salt
- Rub the olive oil on the acorns
- Bake for 45 minutes
- In a saucepan at medium heat, pour in canola oil and onions
- Stir till light and soft
- Pour in broth and leave to simmer on low heat for 15 minutes
- Put in baked acorn, curry, and pepper
- Boil for 15 minutes
- Take off fire and let cool
- Place in blender and blend till smooth
- Serve warm

16. Tomato soup
NUTRITIONAL VALUE PER SERVING

Calories: 270g; Fat: 9g; carbohydrates: 40g; 2.7 g; sugar; 24g
protein: 20.5g

Preparation time: 45 minutes

Ingredients:

- 250g of fresh and firm tomatoes
- Salt to taste
- 1 large onion
- 1 tablespoon of curry
- 1 tablespoon turmeric powder
- 1 teaspoon red pepper
- 200 grams of chicken stock
- 3 teaspoons of canola oil

Directions

- Chop up tomatoes and blend alone. Add little water so it is thick and smooth
- Place large saucepan and heat at medium heat
- Pour in oil and then onions
- Stir fry till onions is soft
- Put in curry and pepper
- Pour in stock and close pot
- Allow to boil for 15 minutes
- When cool, blend again if your mixture is not fully smooth

17. Carrot chicken soup

NUTRITIONAL VALUE PER SERVING

Calories: 120g Fat: 10g ; carbohydrates: 15g; protein: 27g; potassium: 148mg

Preparation time: 1 ½ hours

Ingredients:

- 250g of raw and bone-free chicken, no skin
- ½ teaspoon
- 1 small onion, chopped
- 2 stock cubes
- 1 tablespoon of curry
- 1 tablespoon turmeric powder
- 1 teaspoon red pepper
- 1 bay leaf
- 3 carrots
- 4 cups of water

Directions

- Chop chicken in small pieces
- Next, chop the carrot in small pieces
- Place chicken, salt to, carrot, onions, stock cubes, curry, turmeric, pepper in large saucepan
- Pour in water and place on heat
- Let boil for 45 minutes
- When boiled take out chunks of carrot and meat and blend till roughly. Do not let it get smooth
- Put back in pot and boil let simmer on low heat for 3 hours
- Strain to take out all particles

Sample meal plan for stage 1 gastric bypass surgery

You are expected to take liquids every two hours. You should not take more than two ounces at a go.

- 07:00am- 08:00am[part 1]: 7-8 ounces of carrot chicken soup
- 09:00am- 10:00am[part 2]: 7- 8 ounces of water
- 11:00am- 01:00pm[part 3]: 7- 8 ounces of carrot chicken soup
- 02:00pm- 03:00pm[part4]:7-8 8ounces of carrot chicken
- 04:00pm- 05:00pm [part 5]:7- 8 ounces of carrot chicken soup
- 06:00pm- 07:00pm[part 6]: 7- 8 ounces of water
- 08:00pm- 09:00pm[part 7]: 7- 8 ounces of carrot chicken soup

Remember to take about 1- 15 minutes on each ounce. Take your time. The meal plan is also flexible. In one stage, you can have 4 ounces of two different types of clear liquids or 3.5 each. If you feel it is too much for your body, you may spread out 48 ounces. Remember not to try more than one new food in a day. When you have tried foods, you can start to mix.
Remember to check calorie counts. If a serving has much more calories than you need, you can get half or a quarter.

Stage 2A- Full liquids meal plan

This stage is the bridge between clear liquids and purred food. It is done this way so you do not end up rushing your body. You do not have to strain most of your food anymore. You must remember not to rush your body. It is from here that you will begin to eat six times daily.

Stage 2A- Full liquids recipes

18. Liquid cooked oats and skimmed milk
NUTRITIONAL VALUE PER SERVING

Calories: 230.9g Fat: 2g; Cholesterol: 18.0 mg; Sodium: 60.8 mg; Potassium: 1.8 mg; Total Carbohydrate: 32.5 g; Dietary Fiber: 7.0 g; Sugars: 6.5 g; Protein :9.1 g

Preparation time: 30 minutes

Ingredients:

- ½ cup of Quaker oats
- ½ cup of water
- 1 cup of skimmed milk

Directions

- Pour in oats into a small bowl and put in water to the exact level of the oats
- Cover and leave for 20 minutes
- The oats should absorb the water
- Pour in the soaked oats in a sauce pan
- Put in the cup of skimmed milk
- Put it on a low heat and let it simmer till it becomes thick.
- Serve warm

19. Sugar free light yogurt
NUTRITIONAL VALUE PER SERVING

Calories: 50g Fat: 2g; Cholesterol: 11mg; Sodium: 36mg; Potassium: 1.8 mg; Total Carbohydrate: 10g; Sugars: 7g; Protein :3g

Preparation time: 30 minutes

Ingredients:

- 1 cup grapes
- ¼ cup of Silk Dairy-Free Almond yogurt

Directions

- Steam grapes in for five minutes in *very little* water
- Turn water and grapes in a cup and remove the skin
- Freeze grapes and complete water
- Blend the grapes until they are halfway smooth
- Put of blender and pour in yoghurt
- Blend well until smooth
- Freeze and enjoy cold

20. Coconut creamy acorn soup

NUTRITIONAL VALUE PER SERVING

Calories: 250g; Fat: 10g; cholesterol: 1mg; pottasium:992mg; carbohydrates: 29g; 2.7 g fiber: 4g; sugar; 2g protein: 4g

Preparation time: 1 ½ hours

Ingredients:

- 2 tablespoons of olive oil 1 large sliced onion
- 3 acorn squashes [cut and seeded]
- 2 tablespoons of olive oil
- 1 cup of chicken broth
- ½ cup of coconut milk
- 1 tablespoon of ground curry
- 1 basil leaf
- Pinch of salt

Directions

- Cut each acorn squash in half and seed
- Preheat oven to 400 degrees F
- Line a baking sheet and placed it acorns face down on it
- Mix olive oil with a pinch salt
- Rub the olive oil on the acorns
- Bake for 45 minutes
- In a saucepan at medium heat, pour in olive oil and onions
- Stir till soft
- Pour in broth and leave to simmer on low heat for 15 minutes
- Boil for 15 minutes
- While it is boiling, put in milk in a bowl and put in baked acorn squashes

- After 15 minutes, place them in blender and blend till smooth
- Take off fire and let cool
- Serve warm

21. *Chicken peanut apple sauce*

NUTRITIONAL VALUE PER SERVING

Calories: 50 kal; Fat: 2 grams; Cholesterol: 0.060 grams; Sodium: 0.203 grams; Carbohydrates: 13 grams; Dietary Fiber: 2 grams; Sugar: 10 grams; Protein: 3 grams.

Preparation time: 1 ½ hours

Ingredients:

- 3 pounds of chicken pieces
- ¼ cups of mustard
- ⅛ cups of brown sugar
- ⅛ cups of brown sugar
- ½ cups of peanuts (powdered)
- Salt (To taste)
- Pepper (as desired)
- 1 jar of unsweetened applesauce
- Water

Directions

- Defreeze your chicken ahead if needed
- Wash the chicken thoroughly
- Place chicken in a sauté pan with water and cook on medium heat.
- When it is almost completely cooked, add apple sauce, mustard, brown sugar and the powdered peanuts.
- Stir well to achieve uniformity.
- Continue to cook over medium heat until it is 75°c hot
- Let it down after 5 minutes
- Serve warm

22. Soy dessert

NUTRITIONAL VALUE PER SERVING

Calories: 56 kal; Carbohydrate: 6 grams; unsaturated Fat: 1 gram; Protein: 5 grams; Cholesterol: 0.001 grams; Sodium: 0.181 grams

Preparation time: 15 minutes

Ingredients:

- 1 envelope of Knox original unflavored gelatin
- 1/3 cup of boiling water
- 1 package (1.4 ounces)of sugar-free, fat-free chocolate fudge instant pudding (Preferably Jell-o)
- 1 ½ cups of cold skimmed milk
- 16 ounces of silken tofu
- ½ teaspoon of vanilla extract
- 2 tablespoons of cocoa powder
- ¼ teaspoons of peppermint extract

Directions

- Mix the boiling water and unflavored gelatin into a small bowl.
- Set the mixture aside and allow it to coagulate.
- Chop the Tofu finely and place it into the pudding mixture. Whisk quickly and vigorously to break up the soy cubes
- Add in the vanilla and peppermint extracts alongside the cocoa powder
- Transfer the mixture into a blender/ food processor and Blend until the mixture is smooth and consistent. Shake the contents every 5 seconds or use your hands to mix it. This will ensure that the pudding does not make the blender motor stick.

- The mixture should now resemble a smoothie in its texture. Gradually add gelatin and stir until they are well combined.
- Blend for another 5 minutes
- Pour the mixture into a glass dish, cover and place into a refrigerator.
- Leave to chill for at least1 hour
- Cut into 8 portions and serve

23. Crockpot oatmeal
NUTRITIONAL VALUE PER SERVING

Calories: 139 kals; Serving size: 20 (1/2 cup servings); Protein: 6.35; Carbohydrates: 1.91; Fat: 4.(all in grams)

Preparation time: 15 minutes

Ingredients:

- 2 cups of oats
- 2 teaspoons of cinnamon
- 10 cups of water
- 4 ounces of dried cranberries
- ½ teaspoon of salt
- 4 ounces of raisins
- 4 ounces of slivered almonds
- 1 tablespoon of stevia

Directions

- Place the water in a small pot
- Wash your raisins and almonds in clean water
- Add in the oats, dried cranberries, raisins, almonds, Stevia and salt.
- Set to high heat and cook for 180 minutes
- Add cinnamon then stir
- Serve in bowls
- Top oats with either two tablespoons of Greek yogurt (fat free) or soy yogurt

24. Chicken cauliflower
NUTRITIONAL VALUE PER SERVING

Calories: 236 kal; Carbohydrate: 16 grams; unsaturated Fat: 9 gram; Protein: 13 grams; Cholesterol: 0.1 grams; Sodium: 0.181 grams

Preparation time: 15 minutes

Ingredients:

- 1 head of a cauliflower
- 3 garlic cloves
- ¼ cup chicken broth
- ¼ cup plain Greek yogurt
- 1 tablespoon canola oil
- ½ teaspoon of black pepper
- 2 medium-sized diced onions
- Salt

Directions

- Chop up the cauliflower
- Peel and slice garlic
- In a pot, bring water to boil
- Put in cauliflower in a pot
- Place in garlic and a pinch of salt
- Cover for 7 minutes
- Take out cauliflower and place them in 4 layers of paper towel
- Squeeze them out to get out all the water
- If the towels are not enough, use more
- Place them in a processor add broth, yoghurt, pinch of salt, and oil
- Process until smooth

Sample meal plan for stage 2A gastric bypass surgery

- 07:00am- 07:30am[part 1]: 8 ounces of water
- 08:00am- 9:00am[part 2]: protein shake
- 09:30am- 11:30pm[part 3]: 12 ounces of chicken cauliflower soup
- 12:00pm- 01:00pm[part4]: snack such as ½ cup of cottage cheese
- 01:00pm- 03:00pm [part 5]:2 servings of chicken peanut apple sauce [or something up to 100 kals]
- 03:30pm- 04:00pm[part 6]: 12 ounces of water
- 04:30pm- 06:00pm[part 7]: snack such as Greek yogurt
- 06:30pm- 07:30pm[part 6]: 8 ounces of water
- 09:00pm- 09:30pm[part 7]: 8 ounces of carrot chicken soup

On the first day of stage 2A, consume around

- Calories: 470
- Protein: 66g
- Fluids: 60 oz

On the second day of stage 2A, consume around

- Calories: 530
- Protein: 69g
- Fluids: 60 oz

On the third day of stage 2A, consume around

- Calories: 600
- Protein: 68g
- Fluids: 56 oz

You can maintain this, plus or minus
Remember to check calorie counts. If a serving has much more calories than you need, you can get half or a quarter.

Stage 2B- Pureed foods meal plan

Pureed foods are high in protein and can easily be mashed. You should be taking up to 60 to70 grams of protein and 64 ounces of fluids water. Your food must be very moist and remember not to mix fluids with meals. Give them a 30 minutes gap. If you do not chew extremely slowly and thoroughly, you will vomit. Go easy on yourself and only try one new food daily. Do not eat raw fruits or vegetables yet.

Stage 2B- Pureed foods recipes

25. Peanut powder salad dressing
NUTRITIONAL VALUE PER SERVING

Calories: 50 kals; Carbohydrates grams: 7; Sodium: 0.563 grams; Fat: 2 grams; Protein:3 grams ; Dietary Fiber: 1.21 grams ; Sugar: 5 grams

Preparation time: 20 minutes

Ingredients:

- 1/2 tablespoon of soy sauce
- 1/2 tablespoon of water
- 1 tablespoon of peanut powder
- 1/4 teaspoon of garlic powder
- 1/2 teaspoon of ground pepper
- 1/2 teaspoon of Szechuan chili sauce
- 2 teaspoons of brown sugar blend
- 1/2 teaspoon of sesame oil

Directions

- Pour all the ingredients into a blender or food processor and blend until a smoothie like consistency is gotten. This should take 10 approximately 10 minutes.
- Serve and refrigerate any remaining sauce.

26. Egg chilada
NUTRITIONAL VALUE PER SERVING

Calories: 171kals; Sugar: 3 grams; Carbohydrate:3 grams; Protein: 23 grams , Fat:8 grams

Ingredients:

- 1 full egg
- 1 egg white
- 1 ounce of chicken
- 2 tablespoons of Salsa
- Black pepper
- 2 tablespoons Mexican cheese (shredded)
- 3 tablespoons of plain fat-free Greek yoghurt
- Salt to taste

Directions

- Defreeze chicken
- Place both egg and egg white in a bowl and whisk briskly
- Pour your whisked eggs into a preheated pan. Let the circumference cover the whole pan evenly
- Sprinkle your salt and pepper as the eggs begin to harden
- Flip the eggs (Use a spatula to help if it is stuck the pan) to enable the other side cook as well
- Take out the eggs and lay flat
- Fill the eggs with spoonfuls of chicken and Mexican cheese.
- Roll up the eggs
- Top with Greek yogurt and salsa

27. Moist chicken
NUTRITIONAL VALUE PER SERVING

Calories: 233 kal; Sugar 0g; Carbohydrate: 8g; Fat: 5g; Protein: 37g; Sodium: 268mg

Preparation time: 55 minutes

Ingredients:

- 3 ½ pounds skinned chicken breasts (boneless)
- 1 and 1/3 Italian bread crumbs (whole wheat)
- 1½ jar of light mayonnaise dressing

Directions

- Preheat your oven to a temperature of about 420 °
- Apply mayonnaise over the total surface of the pieces of chicken breasts
- Place your breadcrumbs in a large and flat tray and roll the soaked chicken parts through it
- Place foil on a pan and bake the crumb covered chicken for 45-50 minutes

28. Creamy tarragon dressing
NUTRITIONAL VALUE PER SERVING

Per half cup serving: Calories: 189kal; protein 11.17g; Carbohydrate: 19.166g; Fat 7.25g.

Preparation time: 15 minutes

Ingredients:

- 1 Tablespoon fresh minced tarragon
- 1 tablespoon of spicy mustard (brown)
- ½ cup of plain yogurt (fat free)
- ¼ cup no fat sour cream
- ¼ cup of apple juice concentrate (unsweetened)

Directions

- In a bowl, put in tarragon and yoghurt
- Pour in mustard and mix
- Put in sour cream and mix
- Then put in apple juice and mix
- Serve

29. Steam fish and yogurt sauce

Calories: 270 kals; Fat: 6 g; saturated fat:1 g; cholesterol: 95 mg; protein: 46 g; calcium: 20mg; sugars: 9g

Preparation time: 15 minutes

Ingredients:

- ½ cup low-fat, plain yogurt
- 1 diced scallion include the green part
- 1 large lemon, thinly sliced
- ½ cup of chicken broth
- 2 tablespoons canola oil
- 1 teaspoon finely chopped fresh basil
- 1 ½ pounds of firm-fleshed salmon
- 1 tablespoon of divided fresh dill
- 1 tablespoon finely chopped fresh chives
- Salt to taste
- Pepper to taste

Directions

- Put oil, salt, basil, chives and half of the dill
- Mix together and rub the fish with it
- Pour yogurt in a bowl and put in dill. Cover and set aside
- Mix remaining dill with yogurt and set sauce aside.
- Place scallions in large rimmed dish
- Place fish on scallions
- Place lemon in slices on the fish
- Pour in broth
- Microwave till soft and serve with yoghurt

30. Refried kidney beans
NUTRITIONAL VALUE PER SERVING

Calories: 253 kals; Fat: 11 g; saturated fat:1 g; cholesterol: 45 mg; protein: 56 g; calcium: 36mg;

Preparation time: 15 minutes

Ingredients:

- 1 can kidney beans

Directions

- Dice onions
- Set a saucepan on medium heat
- Open up can of beans and pour in with the water
- Add onions, garlic, cumin, salt and pepper
- Cook until it boils well
- Take off and leave to cool
- Mash and reheat
- If it is too thick, you can put in vegetable stock

31. Black bean soup
NUTRITIONAL VALUE PER SERVING

Calories: 273 kals; Fat: 13 g; saturated fat:1 g; cholesterol: 48.5 mg; protein: 65 g; calcium: 36mg;

Preparation time: 15 minutes

Ingredients:

- 1 can of black beans
- ½ teaspoon chili powder
- 1 teaspoon cumin
- 1 minced garlic clove
- 1 teaspoon minced jalapeños
- 1 teaspoon tomato paste
- Kosher salt
- Black pepper
- 8 ounces of vegetable stock
- 1 bay leaf
- Sour cream
- 1 tablespoon canola oil

Directions

- Heat oil in saucepan over medium heat
- Put in onions and fry till soft
- Add jalapeños and then garlic
- Stir fry for 2-3 minutes
- Put in tomato paste
- Add salt, pepper, chili and cumin
- Stir well
- Open can and pour in beans with the water in them
- Add bay leaf and leave to boil on low heat for 15-20 minutes
- Take off heat and allow to cool
- Using blender or food processor, blend food till it is as smooth as you want

Sample meal plan for stage 2B gastric bypass surgery

- 07:00am- 07:30am[part 1]: 8 ounces of water
- 08:00am- 9:00am[part 2]: protein shake
- 09:30am- 11:30pm[part 3]: snack such as Greek yogurt
- 12:00pm- 01:00pm[part4]: 8 ounces of water
- 01:00pm- 03:00pm [part 5]: 2 ounces peanut powder salad dressing
- 03:30pm- 04:00pm[part 6]: 1 serving refried kidney beans
- 04:30pm- 06:00pm[part 7]: 3 ounces Steam fish and yogurt sauce
- 06:30pm- 07:30pm[part 6]: 12 ounces of water
- 09:00pm- 09:30pm[part 7]: sugar-free jello

On the first day of stage 2B, consume around

- Calories: 500
- Protein: 60-70g
- Fluids: 60 -64oz

On the second day of stage 2B, consume around

- Calories: 550
- Protein: 65-70g
- Fluids: 60-64 oz

On the third day of stage 2, consume around

- Calories: 650
- Protein: 70g
- Fluids: 60-64 oz

You can maintain this, plus or minus

Remember to check calorie counts. If a serving has much more calories than you need, you can get half or a quarter.

Stage 3- Soft foods meal plan

Here you can begin to take real foods that are soft. You must still chew meticulously. Don't eat more than one new food daily. If your body reacts negatively to a food, take note of it and wait 3 weeks before trying it again cautiously.

You must eat 3 servings fruits and vegetables per day. You must also have 3 servings of whole grains per day; that is ½ of a cup. Lastly, you should have 8-10 grams of fiber per day.

You should also have 6 meals; breakfast, snack or fluid, lunch, snack or fluid, dinner, and snack or fluid.

Try new foods each day so you can have a wide variety

Stage 3- Soft foods recipes

32. Pineapple meatballs
NUTRITIONAL VALUE PER SERVING

Serving size: 24(2 each) meatballs; Calories: 91 kals; Protein: 6.43 grams; Carbohydrates: 13.37 grams; Fat: 1.3 grams.

Preparation time: 30 minutes

Ingredients:

- 2cans of pineapple chunks
- 1 cup of chopped bell pepper
- 2 tablespoons light soy sauce
- 24 pairs of turkey meatballs
- 4 tablespoons of corn starch
- 4 beef bouillon cubes

Directions:

- Place all ingredients (except the corn starch) together in a pot.
- Boil gently for 17 minutes
- Pour some water into the cornstarch
- Stir until it's even, thick and clear.
- Place the meatballs into it
- Boil gently for 12 minutes
- Serve warm

33. Baked tomatoes
NUTRITIONAL VALUE PER SERVING

Calories: 73kals; Sugar: 3 grams; Carbohydrate: 6 grams;
Protein: 3 grams ; Fat:5 grams; Dietary fiber: 2 grams

Preparation time: 1 ½ hours

Ingredients

- 8 small fresh tomatoes
- Extra virgin olive oil cooking spray
- ½ cups of shredded low fat parmesan cheese
- Greek Seasoning
- Salt

Directions

- Oven must be preheated to 177° c.
- Wash and half each tomato
- Place each half face down on a non-stick frying pan
- Rub the outer covering of each tomato with the extra virgin olive oil
- Coat with pine nuts and cheese (The oil will help it stick)
- Sprinkle a pinch of salt
- Place in the preheated oven and let it bake for 50 minutes.

34. High protein cheesecake
NUTRITIONAL VALUE PER SERVING

Calories: 152 kal; Sugar 2g; Carbohydrate: 610g; Unsaturated Fat: 7g; Protein: 13g; Sodium: 385 mg.

Preparation time: 50 minutes

Ingredients:

- ½ teaspoons of baking soda
- 1/3 teaspoons of olive oil
- 1 cup low-fat cottage cheese
- 1 teaspoons of peppermint extract
- 3 large eggs

Directions

- Beat eggs
- Mix your flour and baking powder together in a small bowl
- In a bigger bowl, mix your cottage cheese, eggs, peppermint extract, and olive oil
- Pour the flour mixture into the bigger bowl containing the cheese
- Stir with a spoon until they are thoroughly mixed together
- Set fire to medium heat and place a pan on
- Pour the batter into the pan and cook until bubbles begin to escape. Wait until it hardens a bit
- Flip the batter and repeat the process until both sides have a brownish shade
- May be served with syrup (low calorie)

35. Cake o' watermelon
NUTRITIONAL VALUE PER SERVING

(per one inch slice): Calories: 106kal; protein 3.2g; Carbohydrate: 13.15g; Fat 5.1g.

Preparation time: 30 minutes

Ingredients:

- 1 watermelon (approximately 6 cups)
- 1 packet of vanilla pudding (sugar free)
- 1 container of whipped cream (sugar free)
- 5 inch long bamboo skewers
- 1 cup of slivered pecans(toasted)
- Sliced mixed fruits (berries)
- 1 teaspoon almond flavoring (optional)

Directions

- Slice the watermelon into three equal parts.
- Peel away the outer covering
- Mix the vanilla pudding with the almond flavor (this is optional)
- Top a round of the watermelon with half of the mixed fruit and half of the (flavored) vanilla pudding.
- Repeat the process with the remainder of the mixed fruit and pudding on another watermelon piece
- Keep the pudding in place by passing bamboo skewers through the cake. Cut them to the appropriate size if they exceed the length required.
- Coat the whole cake with whipped cream, sprinkling it with toasted pecans for added flavoring and aesthetics.

36. Chicken salad
NUTRITIONAL VALUE PER SERVING

(per half cup serving): Calories: 169kal; protein 19.88g; Carbohydrate: 11.39g; Fat 4.39g.

Preparation time: 15 minutes

Ingredients:

- 6 ounces of boiled and crumbled chicken
- Half an onion (preferably diced)
- 1 package mixed salad greens
- 3 large hardboiled eggs
- ½ cap full of vinegar
- Light mayonnaise
- Salt and pepper
- One half head of lettuce

Directions

- Chop the lettuce
- Place the chicken in a bowl, then the eggs, salad greens, diced onions, vinegar and lettuce.
- Add mayonnaise to your taste
- Stir together
- Season with salt and pepper to taste

37. Corn salad

Calories: 47kal; protein 1.80g; Carbohydrate: 10.6g; Fat 3g.

Preparation time: 20 minutes

Ingredients:

- 5 ears of fresh corn
- Extra virgin olive oil
- 1 teaspoon Jalapeño pepper
- ½ cup of chopped Jicama
- ¼ teaspoon of salt
- 1 teaspoon Stevia
- ½ teaspoon ground cumin
- ½ cup of red bell pepper (chopped)
- ½ finely chopped red onion
- 8 thinly sliced green onions

Directions

- Place a non- stick skillet over medium heat
- Place chopped jicama and jalapeño in the pan with olive oil
- Stir frequently as it sauté's for 2 minutes
- Add onions into the mix and stir until they mix and the onions lose their redness and become clear in color
- Toss in the red bell pepper and cook till tender
- Finally, add corn, ground cumin and green onions. Sauté for an additional 2 minutes and add Stevia if it is not as sweet as you would like.

38. Mussels and coconut milk
NUTRITIONAL VALUE PER SERVING

Calories: 49kal; protein 60g; Carbohydrate: 27g; Fat 15g; sat fat: 5g; sugar 1g

Preparation time: 20 minutes

Ingredients:

- 500g mussels of mussels be sure to have your fishmonger de-bearded it
- 250ml coconut milk
- 1 small red chili pepper
- Handful coriander
- 2 limes, juiced

Directions

- Chop the coriander and chili separately
- Place sauce pan and heat at medium heat
- Put in mussels and coconut milk simultaneously
- Cook for 2 minutes
- The mussels should have opened and if they haven't, leave for a minute more
- Put in lime juice and coriander
- Leave to boil for 1 minute
- Serve warm

39. Salmon and canola noodles
NUTRITIONAL VALUE PER SERVING

Calories: 344 kal; protein 32g; Carbohydrate: 27g; Fat 10g; sat fat: 2g; sugar 4g
Preparation time: 20 minutes

Ingredients:

- 1 salmon fillet
- 1 tablespoon canola oil
- 1 tablespoon of soy sauce
- 1 garlic clove crushed
- 70g of buckwheat soba noodles
- 1 small red chili
- 2 spring onions

Directions:

- Soak noodles in hot water
- Slice onions
- Slice chili
- Preheat the oven to 200C
- Line a baking tray and spray with low fat baking spray
- Place in the fillets and rub with oil and garlic
- Bake for 8 minutes
- Cook noodles with red chili and spring onions
- Let noodles be soft and transparent
- Serve fish with noodles

40. Green salad
NUTRITIONAL VALUE

Calories: 301 kal; protein 22 g; Carbohydrate: 48 g; Fat 5 g; sat fat:3 g; sugar 6g

Preparation time: 10 minutes

Ingredients:

- 250 grams of puy lentils
- 2 carrots
- 1 tablespoon vinegar
- 1 shallot
- 1 bag kale
- 1 tablespoon of canola coconut oil
- 1 handful parsley
- 3 tablespoons of chopped spring onions
- 1 tablespoon mustard
- 1 small bunch dill
- 2 firm tomatoes

Directions:

- Cook the puy lentis
- Chop the shallot, carrot, kale, parsley, dill, and tomatoes separately
- In a salad bowl, put in a teaspoon of oil and rub the bowl
- Put in the lentils followed by the shallot, carrot, kale, parsley, dill, and tomatoes
- Toss the salad
- Pour in the remaining oil

41. Lentil curry soup

Calories: 199 kal; protein 9 g; Carbohydrate: 25g; Fat 7g; sat fat: 5 g; sugar 6g

Preparation time: 20 minutes

Ingredients:

- 500 grams of red lentils
- 400ml low fat coconut milk
- 400g of firm tomatoes
- 150 grams of spinach
- 1 tbsp olive oil
- 1 medium sized onion
- 1 ½ tablespoons of grated ginger
- 1 tablespoon curry powder
- 1 tablespoon of red pepper
- Salt and pepper to taste

Directions

- Chop the onions
- Grate ginger
- Dice tomatoes
- Heat saucepan at medium heat level
- Put in olive oil and onions
- Put in ginger, salt, curry, and pepper to taste
- Stir fry till onions are almost transparent
- Coconut milk
- Close for a minute on low heat and then pour in tomatoes
- Close and let almost boil then put in a cup of water
- Put in lentils and allow to simmer for 35 minutes
- Put in spinach and leave to boil for 2-4 minutes

42. Chicken and salmon casserole
NUTRITIONAL VALUE PER SERVING

Calories: 515 kal; protein 54g; Carbohydrate: 22 g; Fat 10g; sat fat: 18 g; sugar 12g
Preparation time: 20 minutes

Ingredients:

- 1 tablespoon of canola oil
- 2 chicken breasts
- 50g smoked salmon
- 1 medium onion
- 1 green peppers
- 1 cloves ginger, crushed
- ½ teaspoon of curry
- 1 basil leaf
- 150ml passata

Directions:

- Remove skin on chicken and chop into pieces
- Chop salmon into pieces
- Chop onions and peppers
- Preheat the oven to 160C
- Pour canola oil in pan and heat on medium heat
- Put in onions, peppers, ginger, and chopped salmon
- Stir fry for 8-10 minutes
- Pour in passata
- After 10 seconds put in chicken breasts
- Stir the fish and chicken in the sauce
- Take off heat, put basil leaf in and cover pot
- Place in oven to bake for 1 hour

- Open and stir to the other side and let bake for another hour

43. *Mexican baked turkey*

NUTRITIONAL VALUE PER SERVING

Calories: 600 kal; protein 43 g; Carbohydrate: 32 g; Fat 37 g; sat fat: 9 g; sugar 5g

Preparation time: 20 minutes

Ingredients:

- 200g chopped turkey
- 1 serving cooked brown rice
- 2 tablespoons of chopped cauliflower
- 5 firm tomatoes
- 1 jar chipotle paste
- 60ml red wine vinegar
- 3 garlic cloves, peeled
- 1 tablespoon of minced ginger
- Salt
- 1 stock cube

Directions

- Preheat the oven to 180C
- In a saucepan that can survive oven heat pour in the paste and vinegar
- Put on high heat and when it begins to boil, put in turkey
- Then put in garlic and tomatoes
- Put in garlic, ginger and stir
- Put in salt and stock cube
- Stir again
- Cover pan and place in oven for 2 hours
- When ready, serve with rice

44. Cream soup
NUTRITIONAL VALUE PER SERVING

Calories: 225.7 kal; protein 4.6 g; Carbohydrate: 39 g; Fat 5.7 g;
sat fat: 3 g; sugar 4.4g
Preparation time: 25 minutes

Ingredients:

- 1 cup strained cream soup
- 1 cup smooth mashed potatoes
- A pinch of salt
- ¼ teaspoon of canola oil

Directions:

- In a skillet, pour in cream soup
- Pour in mashed potatoes
- Heat on low heat till it simmers
- Serve warm

45. Cauliflower soup
NUTRITIONAL VALUE PER SERVING

Calories: 214 kal; protein 32g; Carbohydrate: 19g; Fat 12.5g; sat fat: 2g; sugar 3g
Preparation time: 45 minutes

Ingredients

- 1 small cooked cauliflower
- 1 medium sized onion
- 3 teaspoons canola oil
- 4 teaspoons of protein powder
- 2 cups skimmed milk
- 1 teaspoon salt
- 1 egg yolk
- 2 tablespoons of grated low fat mozzarella cheese
- ½ cup of spicy sausage, cooked

Directions

- Shred cauliflower
- Mix cauliflower in milk and set aside
- Heat oil in large skillet
- Pour in onions and stir fry
- Put in protein powder and stir
- Pour in milk and cauliflower
- Allow to simmer
- Take off fire and blend well

46. *Borscht yogurt*

261 calories, 5g total fat, 1g saturated fat, 1mg cholesterol, 581mg sodium, 48g carbohydrate, 10g fiber, 17g sugar, 8g protein,

Preparation time: 20 minutes

Ingredients:

- 2 ½ cups plain low-fat yogurt
- ¾ cups sour cream
- 1/4 tablespoons of salt
- 1/4 tablespoons of celery salt
- 1/4 tablespoons of onion salt
- 1 cup of beetroots

Directions

- Dice and cook the beetroots
- Pour the sour cream, yoghurt, celery salt, onion salt, beets and salt in blender.
- Switch on the blender and blend till mixture is smooth
- Add ice cubes or chill to enjoy.

47. Sweet potato soup
NUTRITIONAL VALUE PER SERVING

Calories: 218 kal; protein 5.62g; Carbohydrate: 35.5g; Fat 6.46g; Sugar :17.1g

Preparation time: 20 minutes

Ingredients

- 1 ½ teaspoon of salt
- 1 ½ cup mashed sweet potatoes
- 1 tablespoon of butter
- 1 of protein powder
- 1 tablespoon of brown sugar
- 1 tablespoon of chicken broth
- 1/4 tablespoon of ginger
- 1/8 tablespoon of cinnamon
- 1 cup of skimmed milk

Directions

- Blend the potatoes, ginger, broth, butter, salt, sugar, cinnamon and protein powder together in the blender.
- Pour into a skillet and stir until mixture comes to a boil
- Reduce heat and leave for about 4 minutes.
- Serve hot.

48. Cream of mushroom soup
NUTRITIONAL VALUE PER SERVING

 Calories: 431.4kal; protein 2.7g; Carbohydrate: 18.9g; Fat 4.9g; sat fat: 0.8g; sugar : 0.6g

Preparation time: 20 minutes

Ingredients

- 6 tablespoons of protein powder
- 2 tablespoons of olive oil
- 2 cans of chicken broth
- ½ pound of mushrooms
- ¼ cup of chopped onion
- ¼ teaspoon of salt
- 1/8 teaspoon of pepper
- 1 cup of whole milk cream

Directions

- Slice the mushrooms and pour into saucepan with onions.
- Over medium heat, Sauté onions and mushrooms in olive oil till they are well cooked.
- Pour one can of chicken broth, protein powder, pepper and salt into one bowl.
- Stir until ingredients are well mixed.
- Pour the mixture into the saucepan with mushrooms and onions.
- Empty the remaining can of chicken broth into the mixture and stir.
- Place over medium heat and bring to a boil while constantly stirring.
- Stir in the cream after about 2 minutes
- Uncover the pot and leave to boil for 15 minutes.

49. *Lobster bisque*
NUTRITIONAL VALUE PER SERVING

Calories 310, calories from fat 210, total fat 24g, saturated fat 15g, trans fat 1g, cholesterol 115mg, total carbohydrate 13g, sugars 1g, protein 12g, calcium 10%, iron 4%.

Preparation time: 20 minutes

Ingredients

- 2 ½ cups of skimmed milk
- 1 tablespoon of protein powder
- 1 tablespoon of canola oil
- 2/3 cup of cooked lobster meat
- 1 tablespoon of salt
- 1/4 tablespoon of paprika
- Dash pepper

Directions

- Blend the protein powder, skimmed milk, pepper, salts, oil, paprika and lobster meat together.
- Over low heat, bring to a boil while stirring.
- Strain of excess moisture.

50. Curried fish bisque
NUTRITIONAL VALUE PER SERVING

Calories: 459 kal; protein 32g; Carbohydrate: 24g; Fat 25;

Preparation time: 25 minutes

Ingredients:

- 1 tablespoon of salt
- Dash of paprika
- Dash of pepper
- 1 tablespoon of protein powder
- 2 ½ cups of skimmed milk
- 1 tablespoon of olive oil
- ¼ tablespoon of curry
- 1 cup of cooked lean white meat fish (NO BONES)

Directions

- Blend protein powder, oil, milk and spices together.
- Put in fish and blend
- Pour the mixture in saucepan
- Heat on low heat for 15-20 minutes

51. Poached eggs salad

72 calories; 4.7 g total fat; 1.6 g saturated fat; 185 mg cholesterol; 149 mg sodium. 69 mg potassium; 0.3 g carbohydrates; 6.3 g protein; 28 mg calcium; 1 mg iron; 6 mg magnesium

Preparation time: 15 minutes

Ingredients:

- 1 egg
- 1 ½ teaspoons of vinegar

Directions

- Crack eggs without piercing yolk
- Boil a little water to about 1.5 to 2 inches height of the pot
- Put in vinegar
- Gently pour the eggs into the boiling water from the bowl
- Cook for 5 minutes
- Serve warm

52. Egg salad

Per Serving: 100 calories; 5.8 g fat; 3.1 g carbohydrates; 8.1 g protein; 212 mg cholesterol; 388 mg sodium

Preparation time: 25 minutes

Ingredients:

- 6 hard boiled eggs
- 1/3 cup low-fat mayonnaise
- 1/3 cup chopped fresh chives
- ½ teaspoon paprika
- ½ teaspoon pepper
- ½ teaspoon Dijon mustard
- ¼ teaspoon pink salt

Directions:

- Cut up 4 or the eggs into chunks
- Take out the eggs of the remaining 2 eggs and cut up only the whites
- Mix all ingredients together
- Serve

53. *Turkey salad*

417 calories; 19.8 g total fat; 3.2 g saturated fat; 70 mg cholesterol; 467 mg sodium. 892 mg potassium; 29.7 g carbohydrates; 2.6 g fiber; 13 g sugar; 31.5 g protein; 34 mg vitamin c; 168 mcg folate; 124 mg calcium; 3 mg iron; 91 mg magnesium; 7 g added sugar;

Preparation time: 25 minutes

Ingredients:

- 6 cups mixed salad greens
- 3 tablespoons dried cranberries
- 3 cups chopped cooked turkey
- 3 tablespoons olive oil
- ½ cup leftover wheat bread stuffing
- ½ cup of protein powder
- ¼ cup cranberry sauce
- 1 tablespoon cider vinegar
- 1 teaspoon grated orange zest
- 1 cup roasted Brussels sprouts
- ¼ teaspoon salt
- ¼ teaspoon black pepper

Directions

- Place skillet with olive oil on medium heat
- Pour in wheat bread stuffing and stir
- Pour in protein powder
- Stir for 3-5 minutes
- Pour in cranberry sauce
- Our in orange zest and stir for a minute

- Put in vinegar and stir
- Put in salt and pepper to taste
- Put in turkey, vegetables and cranberries
- Stir and serve warm

54. Tuna salad
NUTRITIONAL VALUE PER SERVING

Calories: 404 kal; protein 49g; Carbohydrate: 12.5g; Fat 17.5;

Preparation time: 25 minutes

Ingredients:

- 2 cans of tuna
- 1/8 teaspoon mustard
- 1 tablespoon parsley
- Salt and pepper to taste
- 1 minced garlic clove
- 1 small onion
- ½ celery stick
- 1 tablespoon lemon juice

Directions:

- Pour tuna in sieve and drain
- Use a spoon to mash it
- Pour in bowl and put all ingredients except mayonnaise and Dijon
- Mix very well
- Mayonnaise and Dijon mix again and serve

55. Beef stew

317 calories; 9 g total fat; 3.2 g saturated fat; 92 mg cholesterol; 396 mg sodium. 1205 mg potassium; 22.4 g carbohydrates; 4.2 g fiber; 5 g sugar; 35.3 g protein; 7046 IU vitamin a iu; 20 mg vitamin c; 38 mcg folate; 92 mg calcium; 5 mg iron; 65 mg magnesium;

Preparation time:8 hours minutes

Ingredients:

- 3 ounces of red potatoes
- 1 carrot
- 1 small red onion, cut into wedges
- ¼ pound of beef
- 3 ounces of condensed cream of mushroom soup
- 1 cup beef broth
- 1/3 teaspoon of thyme
- 1/3 teaspoon of curry
- 2 ounces of package frozen cut green beans
- 1 stock cube
- ¼ teaspoon salt

Directions

- Quarter the potatoes
- Cut onion into cubes
- Dice carrots
- In a soup pot, pour in potatoes, carrots, onion, beef, mushroom soup, broth, thyme, and curry
- Stir and add stock cube and salt
- Cook on medium heat for 7 hours
- Add green beans
- Cook for 15 minutes
- Serve hot

56. Meatloaf
NUTRITIONAL VALUE

[per serving]Calories: 69 calories; 2.3 g total fat; 0.4 g saturated fat; 19 mg cholesterol; 283 mg sodium. 157 mg potassium; 10.3 g carbohydrates; 1.6 g fiber; 4 g sugar; 2.1 g protein; 420 IU vitamin a iu; 15 mg vitamin c; 13 mcg folate; 20 mg calcium; 1 mg iron; 8 mg magnesium; 1 g added sugar

Preparation time: 1 ½ hours

Ingredients:

- 2 pounds lean ground beef
- ¾ cup dry whole-wheat breadcrumbs
- 2 stalks celery
- 1 onion
- 1 green bell pepper
- 1 tablespoon canola oil
- 4 tablespoons ketchup
- 3 tablespoons Worcestershire sauce
- 1 tablespoon whole-grain mustard
- 1 tablespoon paprika
- 1 teaspoon crushed garlic
- Salt to taste
- Pepper to taste
- 1 egg

Directions

- Chop onions
- Chop celery
- Chop pepper
- Beat egg lightly

- Preheat oven to 375 degrees F
- Spray baking tray with low fat baking spray
- Put in onions, pepper, celery in food processor and make smooth
- Put oil in skillet on medium heat
- Pour in vegetables into pt and stir fry until they are soft
- Take out and let cool
- Add Worcestershire, mustard, garlic, paprika, salt, pepper and half of the ketchup.
- Mix bread an egg crumbs
- Pour in mix
- Put in ground beef
- With your hands mix the mixture
- Spread out the mixture on baking pan
- Pour left over ketchup
- Bake for 45 minutes at 165 degrees F
- Take out and let cool for 15 minutes divide into six servings

57. *Tuna burger*
NUTRITIONAL VALUE

307 calories; 11.8 g total fat; 1.8 g saturated fat; 22 mg cholesterol; 669 mg sodium. 334 mg potassium; 39.1 g carbohydrates; 5.3 g fiber; 7 g sugar; 14.1 g protein; 1315 IU vitamin a iu; 19 mg vitamin c; 34 mcg folate; 67 mg calcium; 2 mg iron; 53 mg magnesium; 5 g added sugar;

Preparation time: 30 minutes

Ingredients:

- 6 ounces light tuna
- 2 slices tomato
- ¼ of cup whole wheat breadcrumbs
- 1/3 cup of low-fat mayonnaise
- 3 tablespoons of roasted red peppers
- ½ stalk of chopped celery
- 3 tablespoons finely chopped onion
- 2 teaspoons extra-virgin olive oil
- 2 whole-wheat hamburger buns or English muffins, toasted
- 2 lettuce leaves
- ½ stock cube

Directions:

- In a large bowl, put in drained tuna
- Pour half of mayonnaise, pepper, and celery
- Sprinkle stock cube and mix well
- The form is to hold together
- Form two patties
- Put in the other half of the mayonnaise and peppers
- Heat oil
- Place molded patties and fry for two minutes on each side
- Spread the mayonnaise and peppers on the top side of each bun.
- Arrange the patty, onions, lettuce and tomato in the bun
- Serve

58. Low fat blackberry yoghurt
NUTRITIONAL VALUE

Calories: 226 kal; protein 11.3g; Carbohydrate: 15g; Fat 3.7;

Preparation time: 15 minutes

Ingredients:

- 2 cups low fat yogurt
- 1 cup blackberries

Directions

- Dice blackberries and freeze
- Pour in yoghurt in food processor
- Put in frozen blackberries process for 5-15 seconds
- Freeze serve cold

59. *Strawberry smoothie*
NUTRITIONAL VALUE

Calories: 154kcal ; Carbohydrates: 30g ; Protein: 8g ; Cholesterol: 2mg ; Sodium: 108mg ; Potassium: 642mg ; Fiber: 4g ; Sugar: 24g ; Vitamin C: 130mg ; Calcium: 278mg ; Iron: 0.9mg

Preparation time: 15 minutes

Ingredients:

- 1 1/3 cup strawberries
- 1 cup crushed ice
- 1/2 cup of non-fat and plain yogurt
- 1 teaspoon lemon juice
- 1 Tablespoon stevia sugar

Directions

- Slice strawberries and freeze
- Take out and set aside
- Place yogurt in blender
- Put in strawberries
- Lemon juice and stevia
- Blend till smooth
- Add ice and serve

60. *Protein banana shake*
NUTRITIONAL VALUE

300 calories, 30 g protein, 11 g fat, 19 g carbs, 4 g fiber

Preparation time: 15 minutes

Ingredients:

- 6 ounces of low fat yogurt
- 2 ½ scoops chocolate flavored protein powder
- 1 banana
- 2 tbsp of natural peanut butter

Directions:

- Chop up banana
- Put in yogurt in blender
- Pour protein powder
- Pour in chopped banana
- Blend for 30 seconds
- Put in peanut butter
- Blend till smooth

Sample meal plan for stage 3 gastric bypass surgery

- 08:00am- 08:30am[Breakfast]: 1 poached egg and ½ slice of wheat bread
- 09:00am- 11:30am[snack/ fluid]: 8 ounces protein shake, 8 ounces of water, 1 cup of skimmed milk
- 12:00pm- 12:30pm[lunch]: 2 servings meat loaf
- 02:00pm- 05:30pm[snack/fluid]: 12 ounces of water, 8 ounces of protein banana shake, 8 ounces of chicken broth
- 06:00pm- 06:30pm [dinner]: 2 ounces peanut powder salad dressing, ¼ cup of strawberries, 1 slice of avocado
- 07:00pm- 10:00pm [snack/fluid]: 12 ounces of water, 1 serving low fat blackberry yogurt, ¼ cup of ricotta cheese

Remember that you should not try more than one new food a day. Also, give 30 minutes space between meals and fluids

On the first day of stage 3, consume around

- Calories: 780
- Protein: 69-75g
- Fluids: 60 -64oz

On the second day of stage 3, consume around

- Calories: 800
- Protein: 73- 75 g
- Fluids: 60-64 oz

On the third day of stage 3, consume around

- Calories: 850
- Protein: 75- 77g
- Fluids: 60-64 oz

You can maintain this, plus or minus

Remember to check calorie counts. If a serving has much more calories than you need, you can get half or a quarter.

Stage 4- Soft foods meal plan

Here is the last stage where you can start eating the way you'll eat for the rest of your life. You must still chew meticulously. Don't eat more than one new food daily. If your body reacts negatively to a food, take note of it and wait 3 weeks before trying it again cautiously. You should also have 6 meals; breakfast, snack or fluid, lunch, snack or fluid, dinner, and snack or fluid. Try new foods each day so you can have a wide variety.

Stage 4- Soft foods recipes

61. Dry cherry and almond scones supreme

Meal type: Snack

Preparation time: 20 mins

NUTRITIONAL VALUE

Serving size: 12 scones; Calories: 133kal; protein 33.48g; Carbohydrate: 11.1g; Fat 5g.

Ingredients:

- 1 egg
- 1 egg white
- 1 scoop of unjury protein powder
- 1 cup of chopped and very dried cherries
- ¼ cup canola oil
- ½ cup granular stevia
- ½ cup low fat butter milk
- ½ teaspoon almond extract
- ½ cup non fat instant powdered milk
- ½ tea spoon baking soda
- 2 cups of wheat flour

Directions

- Preheat your oven to approximately 350 degrees celcius. Try not to exceed this figure
- Apply a non-stick cooking spray on your cookie sheet
- Whisk your eggs and egg white together in a mixing bowl
- Put in butter milk, canola oil, and stevia into separate bowl
- Mix with hand mixer or wooden spoon till well combined
- Pour in eggs and mix again

- Pour in protein powder, powdered milk, and mix well
- Put in wheat flour and mix lightly
- Put in almond extract and mix lightly
- Put in baking soda and mix
- From this, mold out 12 scones
- Lace on lined and sprayed baking sheet and bake for 20-25 minute

62. Gingered ham
Meal type: Lunch

Preparation time: 3 hours

NUTRITIONAL VALUE

Serving size: 8 servings; Calories: 470 kal; protein 63 g;
Carbohydrate: 2g; Fat 23.4g.
Ingredients:

- 6 pounds of boneless gammon joint
- 7 black peppercorns
- 5 cloves
- 3 teaspoons of grated root ginger
- 2 cups of ginger beer; sugar free
- 1 medium onion, diced
- Small root ginger; peeled

Directions

- Slice ginger
- Preheat the oven to 160C or 325F
- Get out roasting pan and spray with low fat baking spray
- Pour in half1 ½ of ginger beer
- Place onions, sliced ginger, cloves, and peppercorns
- Cover with two layers of foil
- Bake for 2 ½ hours be sure to baste once
- Remove and discard all juices
- Set aside
- Increase oven to 200C/400F
- Pour remaining root beer, jam, grated ginger in skillet and let boil

- When it boils reduce heat to low and let the glaze simmer for 6 minutes
- Take off skin from ham. Do not touch the fat layer
- Rub half the glaze on it and bake for another ten minutes without cover
- Take out and rub the rest of the glaze and bake for another ten minutes serve warm

63. *Lamb potato hotpot*
Meal type: Lunch

Preparation time: 20 mins

NUTRITIONAL VALUE

Serving size: 6 servings; Calories: 133kal; protein 32.1g;
Carbohydrate: 29g; Fat 6.2g.
Ingredients:

- 3 bay leaves
- 3 tablespoons oil canola
- 2 onions, thinly sliced
- 2 carrots
- 2 ½ cups of meat stock
- 1 ½ pounds of potatoes
- ½ tablespoon thyme
- 1 ½ pounds of lamb
- 1 tablespoon protein powder
- 1 tablespoon Worcestershire sauce
- Salt and pepper to taste

Directions

- Thinly slice onions and set aside
- Dice lamb and set aside
- Chop carrots and set aside
- Pour in canola oil into oven-safe skillet
- Put in onions, carrot and lam
- Add salt and pepper to taste
- Fry for 5-8 minutes
- Put in protein powder
- Preheat the oven to 200 C/400 F
- Stir fry for 1 minute
- Pour in stock and the Worcestershire sauce
- Cover and let simmer for 15-20 mins
- Slice potatoes into very thin slices
- Place potatoes in stacks in the pots decoratively
- Put in pinch of salt and pepper
- Cover and take off heat
- Place in oven and bake for 1.5 hours
- Take out and place on low heat for thirty minutes

64. Baked chicken and bacon

Meal type: Snack

Preparation time: 1 hour

NUTRITIONAL VALUE

Serving size: 1 serving; Calories: 252 kal; protein 39.7g; Carbohydrate: 4.1g; Fat 8.8g.

Ingredients:

- 4 ounces of chicken; skinless and boneless
- 2 slices of bacon
- ½ teaspoon grated ginger
- ½ teaspoon grated garlic
- 2 teaspoons salsa
- 1 slice tomato
- 1 heaped tbsp grated reduced-fat hard cheese or shredded low-fat mozzarella cheese
- 1 small tomato, sliced
- 2 tablespoons mozzarella cheese
- Salt and pepper to taste

Directions:

- Dice bacon
- Preheat the oven to 190 C/375 F
- Spread out foil and spray low-fat cooking spray
- Put in chicken
- Place bacon all over the chicken at both sides and all over
- Rub garlic and ginger
- Sprinkle salt and pepper
- Wrap tightly
- Leave for 15 minutes
- Unwrap and place in non-stick baking sheet
- Pour pesto sauce over it
- Cover with foil
- Bake for 15 minutes
- Take out and sprinkle cheese
- Place tomatoes
- Bake for 14 minutes

65. *Protein yogurt cookies*

Meal type: Snack

Preparation time: 1 hour

NUTRITIONAL VALUE

Serving size: 12 cookies, 3 servings; Calories: 287; Total Fat: 6g; Total Carbs:4.5g; Protein: 23.8g

Ingredients:

- ¼ cup of protein powder
- ¼ teaspoon baking powder
- 3 eggs
- 5 tablespoons of no fat yogurt

Directions:

- Crack the eggs separate egg whites from the yolk
- Beat the whites till they get bubbly
- Set aside
- In the yolks of the eggs, put in the yoghurt
- Mix well
- Combine both bowl's contents and mix well
- Put in protein powder mix lightly
- Put in baking powder and mix till dough forms
- The result should be somewhat thick
- With a spoon, line out scoops of the baking tray that has parchment
- Lightly spread out the scoops so they are like cookies. They will be very light so apply no pressure
- Bake for 25- 30 minutes
- Take out and leave to cool for an hour

66. *Protein vanilla cookies*
NUTRITIONAL VALUE

Serves 4; Calories: 175; Total Fat: 9g; Total Carbs: 5.5g; Protein: 16.8g
Meal type: Snack

Preparation time: 40 mins

Ingredients:

- 8 tablespoons of low fat cocoa powder
- 1 tablespoon of wheat powder
- 6 tablespoons of canola oil
- 1 flat teaspoon of baking powder
- 2 eggs
- 1 tablespoon confectioners swerve
- 1 1/3 cups of protein powder
- Teaspoon of vanilla extract

Directions:

- Crack and mix the eggs
- Pour eggs in oil to the eggs
- Put in vanilla extract
- Mix very well
- Add cocoa powder
- Add confectioners swerve
- Add protein powder
- Mix very well
- Add baking powder
- Mix till dough forms
- Spread out and cut out your cookies
- Top with the rest of your chocolate chips
- Bake for 8 to 10 minutes
- They will come out very soft
- Set them down and let them cool so they can harden

67. Vanilla frozen yogurt
NUTRITIONAL VALUE

Serves5; Calories: 190; Protein: 60g; Carbs: 14g; Fat: 4.6g

Meal type: Desert

Preparation time: 20 mins

Ingredients:

- ¼ cup of fat-free heavy cream
- 2 tablespoons of stevia
- 1 teaspoon of vanilla extract
- ¾ cup of skimmed milk
- ¾ cup of fat free yogurt

Directions:

- Pour in the vanilla extract and stevia into the blender
- Pour in skimmed milk, fat-free yogurt, and then the heavy cream and blend for 10—20 seconds
- Get out popsicle ice tray
- Pour in liquid, put in possible sticks and freeze

68. Vegan salad dressing

Meal type: Breakfast

Preparation time: 20 mins

NUTRITIONAL VALUE

Serving size: 4; Calories: 58 kal; protein 2 8g; Carbohydrate: 11g; Fat 0g.

Ingredients:

- 2 teaspoons Dijon mustard
- 1/2 cup rice vinegar
- 3 cloves garlic (minced)
- Salt to taste
- Pepper to taste

Directions

- Directions
- Mince garlic
- Pour in mustard, vinegar, garlic, salt, and pepper to taste

69. Shrimp pepper soup

NUTRITIONAL VALUE

Serving size: 2 serving; Calories: 190 kal; protein 25; Carbohydrate: 15 g; Fat 09g.
Meal type: Breakfast

Preparation time: 20 mins

Ingredients:

- 3 ounces fresh shrimp, peeled, cleaned, tails removed
- 1 tablespoon canola oil
- 2 garlic cloves; minced
- 1 clove of minced garlic
- 2 cup of vegetable broth
- 1 tablespoon soy sauce
- 1/2cup baby spinach
- 1 tablespoon lemon juice
- 1 tablespoon chopped parsley

Directions:

- Heat canola oil in skillet on medium heat
- Pour in garlic and ginger
- Stir fry till brown
- Pour in broth, and soy sauce
- Boil and add shrimp
- Let shrimps boil for 3 minutes
- Put in lemon juice and spinach
- Sprinkle parsley and serve

70. Beef canola burger

Meal type: Breakfast/ Lunch

Preparation time: 20 mins

NUTRITIONAL VALUE

Fat: 19g; Carbohydrates: 9g; Calories: 687 kal; Protein: 39g

Ingredients:

- 2 pounds of lean ground beef
- 2 tablespoons canola oil
- 2 cloves of garlic, minced
- 3 tablespoons Worcestershire sauce
- 1 teaspoon of black pepper
- 1 tablespoon of salt

Directions:

- In a bowl pour in the meat, sauce, pepper, and garlic and 2 spoons of oil
- Sprinkle in salt to taste.
- Mix the ingredients very well
- Pour out the mixture on a clean board and mold into patties.
- Place on a grill. Cook each side for around seven minutes
- You can eat with wheat buns

Sample meal plan for stage 4 gastric bypass surgery

- 08:00am- 08:30am[Breakfast]: 2 servings vegan and ½ slice of wheat bread
- 09:00am- 11:30am[snack/ fluid]: 8 ounces protein shake, 8 ounces of broth, 1 cup of skimmed milk
- 12:00pm- 12:30pm[lunch]: 1 serving shrimp pepper soup and avocado slice
- 02:00pm- 05:30pm[snack/fluid]: 12 ounces of water, 8 ounces of protein banana shake, 8 ounces of chicken broth
- 06:00pm- 06:30pm [dinner]: 2 ounces peanut powder salad dressing, ¼ cup of blueberries, 1 slice of avocado
- 07:00pm- 10:00pm [snack/fluid]: 12 ounces of water, 1 serving low fat blackberry yogurt, 2 vanilla cookies

Remember that you should not try more than one new food a day. Also, give 30 minutes space between meals and fluids

On the first day of stage 3, consume around

- Calories: 780
- Protein: 69-75g
- Fluids: 60 -64oz

On the second day of stage 3, consume around

- Calories: 800
- Protein: 73- 75 g
- Fluids: 60-64 oz

On the third day of stage 3, consume around

- Calories: 850
- Protein: 75- 77g
- Fluids: 60-64 oz

You can maintain this, plus or minus

Remember to check calorie counts. If a serving has much more calories than you need, you can get half or a quarter.

Please consult your doctor for dieting pre and after surgery.

Conclusion

If you enjoyed this book and found some benefit in reading it, I'd like to hear from you and hope that you could take some time to post a review on Amazon. Your feedback and support will help this author to greatly improve his writing craft for future projects and make this book even better.

Mike Basso

Made in the USA
Middletown, DE
09 October 2020